# Sensei Self Development

## Mental Health Chronicles Series

*Exploring Your Personal
Goals and Dreams*

Sensei Paul David

# Copyright Page

Sensei Self Development -
Exploring Your Personal Goals and Dreams,
by Sensei Paul David

Copyright © 2024

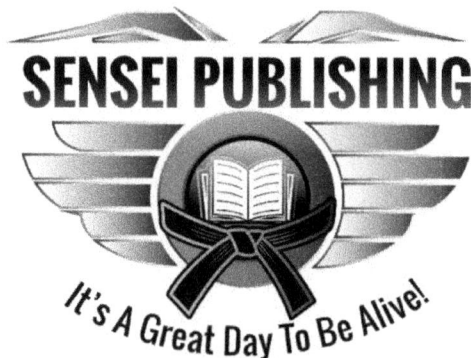

**SENSEI PUBLISHING**

*It's A Great Day To Be Alive!*

www.senseipublishing.com

@senseipublishing
#senseipublishing

# Get/Share Your FREE SSD Mental Health Chronicles at
## www.senseiselfdevelopment.care

### or

## CLICK HERE

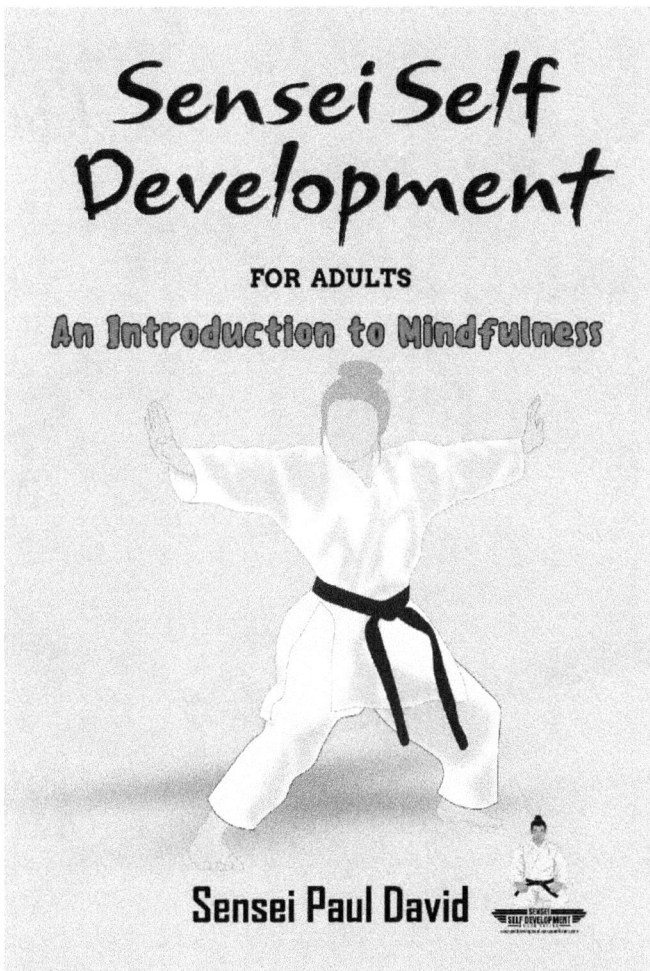

# Check Out The SSD Chronicles Series CLICK HERE

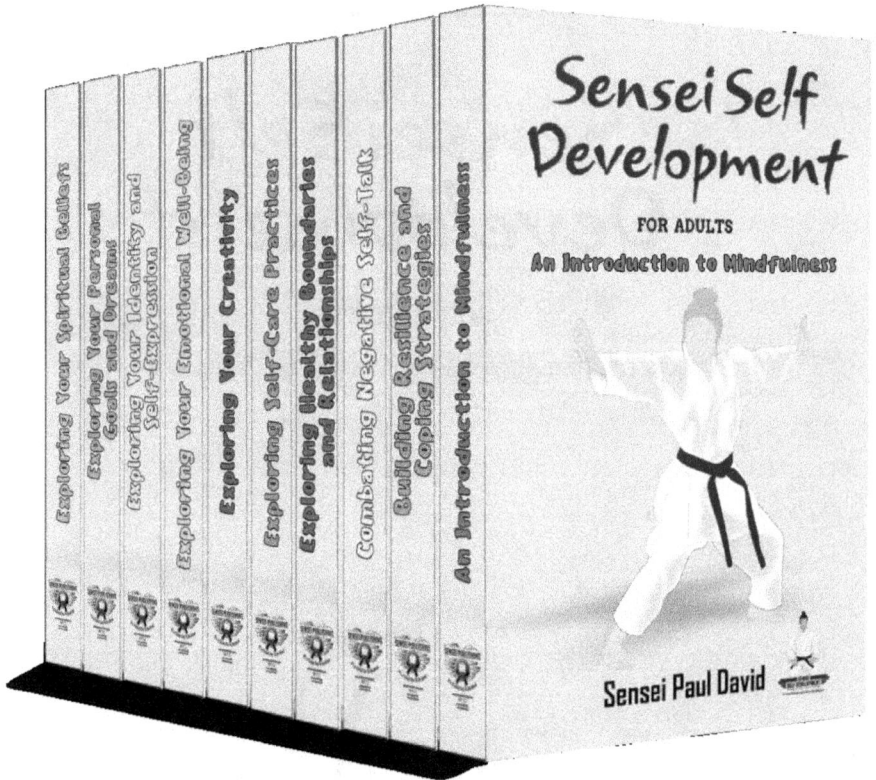

Exploring Your Spiritual Beliefs

Exploring Your Personal Goals and Dreams

Exploring Your Identity and Self-Expression

Exploring Your Emotional Well-Being

Exploring Your Creativity

Exploring Self-Care Practices

Exploring Healthy Boundaries and Relationships

Combatting Negative Self-Talk

Building Resilience and Coping Strategies

An Introduction to Mindfulness

## Sensei Self Development

FOR ADULTS

An Introduction to Mindfulness

Sensei Paul David

# Dedication

To those who courageously take action towards self-improvement - you are helping to evolve the world for generations to come.

- It's a great day to be alive!

# If Found Please Contact:

_____

# Reward If Found:

_____

# MY COMMITMENT

I, _____
commit to writing This Sensei Self
Development Journal for at least 10 days in a
row, starting: _____

Writing this journal is valuable to me because:

_____

_____

_____

_____

_____

_____

If I finish a minimum of 10 consecutive days of
writing in this journal, I will reward myself by:

_____

_____

_____

_____

_____

_____

If I don't finish 10 days of writing this journal, I
will promise to:

_____

_____

_____

_____

_____

_____

I will do the following things to ensure that I
write in my Sensei Self Development Journal
every day:

_____

_____

_____

_____

_____

_____

# Get/Share Your FREE All-Ages Mental Health eBook Now at

www.senseiselfdevelopment.com

## Or CLICK HERE

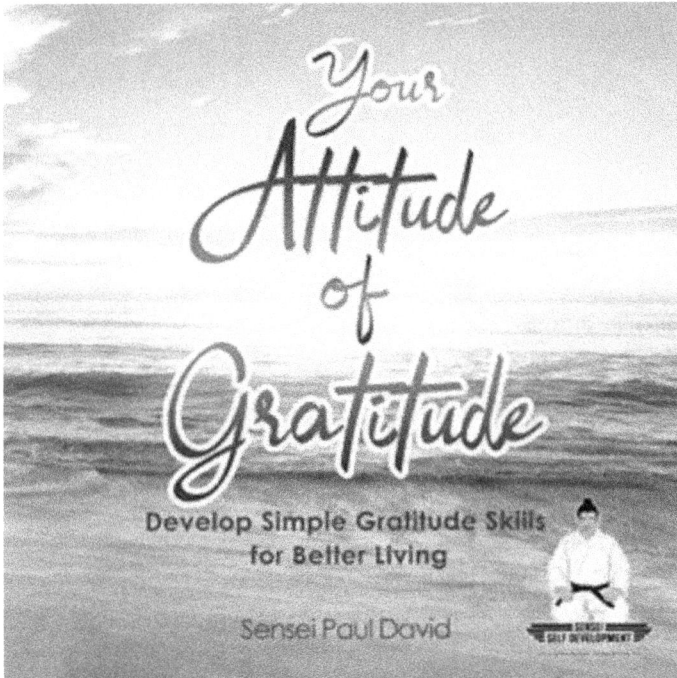

senseiselfdevelopment.com

# Check Out Another Book In The
# SSD BOOK SERIES:

senseipublishing.com/SSD_SERIES

## CLICK HERE

SENSEI
SELF DEVELOPMENT
BOOKS SERIES

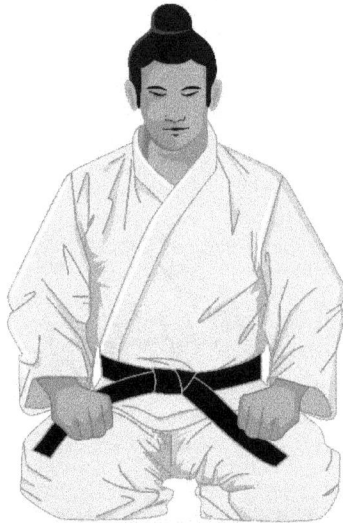

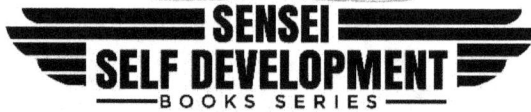

senseiselfdevelopment.senseipublishing.com

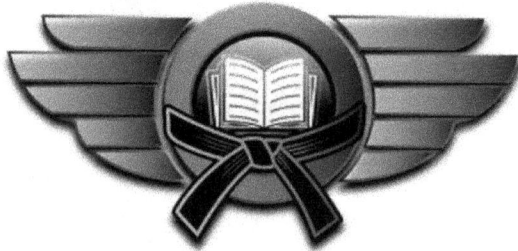

# Join Our Publishing Journey!

If you would like to receive FUTURE FREE BOOKS and get to know us better, please click www.senseipublishing.com and join our newsletter by entering your email address in the pop-up box.

**Follow Our Blog: senseipauldavid.ca**

Follow/Like/Subscribe: Facebook, Instagram, YouTube: @senseipublishing

Scan the QR Code with your phone or tablet

to follow us on social media: Like / Subscribe / Follow

## A Message From The Author:
## Sensei Paul David

Dear Reader,

Welcome to the world of mental health journaling – a sacred space for self-reflection, growth, and healing. Within these pages, you hold the power to uplift your spirit, invigorate your mind, and nourish your goals.

In a world that often moves at blink-and-you'll-miss-it speed, it's crucial to make time for self-care and self-discovery.

Anxiety, stress, and emotional turbulence may have clouded your mind, making it difficult to find clarity and peace within. But fear not! Together, we will navigate the labyrinth of emotions, and experiences, helping to simplify the path to mental well-being.

This journal is not merely a bunch of blank pages awaiting your words. It is your compassionate companion, offering solace and understanding during your unique journey. Here, you are free to unburden yourself, celebrate small and large victories, and confront the challenges that may still linger.

Within the sheltered realm of these pages, there is no judgment, no expectation, and no pressure. Your unique experience and perspective hold immeasurable worth, and your voice deserves to be heard. Whether you choose to fill the lines with eloquence or simply scribble fragments of your thoughts, please remember each entry is a valuable contribution to your growth.

In this sacred space, you are challenged to take off the mask we so often wear in the outside world. It is here that you can be raw, vulnerable, and authentic – allowing your true self to be seen and embraced without reservation. By giving yourself permission to explore the depths of your emotions and confront the shadows that may lurk within, you will discover profound insights and find the healing you seek over time.

As you embark on this journaling journey, I encourage you to embrace the process itself rather than fixate solely on the outcome. Remember, it is not about reaching a certain destination or ticking off boxes on a list of accomplishments. Rather, it is about cultivating self-awareness, fostering self-compassion, and nurturing a sense of curiosity about the intricate workings of your intelligently beautiful mind.

In the quiet moments of reflection, let your pen become a bridge between your inner world and the possibilities that lie ahead. Create a sanctuary for your thoughts, fears, triumphs, and dreams. As you pour your heart onto these pages, allow your words to be a living testament to courage, resilience, and an unwavering commitment to your own well-being.

I am honored to be a part of your journey, and I believe in your ability to navigate the twists and turns with grace and resilience. Remember, you are not alone in this – countless others have walked similar paths, faced similar challenges, and emerged stronger and wiser on the other side. You have the power to reclaim all of your untapped joy, cultivate a positive mindset that serves you, and foster a deep sense of self-love and peaceful confident. – And it will take a worth effort and time.

So, open the first page of this journal with hope, curiosity, and an open heart and open mind. Embrace the transformative power of self-reflection, and allow it to guide you towards a life of greater fulfilment and peace. Each journaling session is an opportunity to not only connect with yourself but also to rekindle the light within that sometimes flickers but never extinguishes.

Remember, the pages you are about to fill are not just a record of your journey but also a testament to your strength, resilience, and indomitable spirit. Cherish this space, invest in yourself, and let your words be an ode to the magnificent journey of becoming whole.

With great respect for your decision to evolve,

Paul

# MY CONVICTION

*Please circle your answers below*

I am DECIDING to be patient with myself and this PROCESS each time I journal toward my improved state of mental well-being

YES        NO

"The present moment is filled with joy and happiness. If you are attentive, you will see it."

*Thich Nhat Hanh*

# Introduction

Happy New Year! Now that the holiday festivities are over and the Christmas tree is off to recycling, it's a good time to start planning for the year ahead. Last year had its challenges, both in the broader world and personally, making it tough to stay on track. But that's okay. This year, you're switching things up by setting goals instead of making resolutions. Choose goals that are measurable and have deadlines, so you can monitor your progress. Apps can help keep you organized and even let you share your progress on social media. A bit of public gloating can boost your motivation (unless, of course, cutting down on social media time is one of your goals.)

To achieve these goals, think about adopting a strategy. For instance, if you want to go to the gym more, set a cue (like keeping your sneakers by the door) and a reward for following through (like a small treat). This way, you're creating a habit loop for yourself.

But, as the year moves on, it's common to hit a slump, especially around February. Don't be discouraged if you start to lose a bit of steam; it's a normal part of the process.

However,

We must make sure that this train, carrying your goals and your dreams, does not screech to a halt. This is what we will learn to do. So, let's start right away.

## How to Set Goals

Every year, it's the same story: We set ambitious New Year's resolutions, broad and lofty. Usually, within a couple of weeks, we stray off course, and by the end of January, those resolutions are long forgotten.

This year, let's switch it up. Let's set resolutions that we can actually stick to.

We usually fail because our resolutions are shaped by what others—society, friends—think we should do, not what we truly want. Also, our goals are often too broad and lack specific, achievable steps. Plus, we tend to aim too high, rather than being realistic.

So, what's the best approach to setting goals if you're serious about making a change? Get S.M.A.R.T about it:

- Specific: Define your goals clearly. Know exactly what you're aiming for and how you'll recognize success.
- Measurable: Find a way to monitor your progress. Whether it's a small daily action or a bigger long-term goal, having some form of measurement helps.
- Achievable: Aim high but stay realistic. Your goal should push you, but still be something you can feasibly achieve.
- Relevant: Pick a goal that really matters to you. You're more likely to persist with something that holds personal value.

- Time-bound: Set a deadline for yourself, and break down your goal into smaller, manageable stages to celebrate as you progress.

## How to Find Your Goal or Dream

You've got a secret. There's something you're keeping to yourself, something only a few, as your partner, your best buddy, or a sibling might know. But to the rest of the world? It's unknown.

You have this dream, something you've wanted to do for the longest time. It's been there, under your skin, like a stubborn splinter you can't quite get rid of. At first, it was tough to even explain. It was more of a gut feeling than anything.

This is about that thing you never talk about.

It's the thing that keeps you awake, staring at the ceiling at night. It's what you daydream about or do when nobody's watching. It's the job or life you really wanted when you were little, not the one you said you wanted to your folks or teachers. Whether it's being a firefighter, an artist, an actor, a globetrotter, or a vet - that's the real you.

A lot of us have lost track of this thing. We've hidden it under retirement plans, health insurance, and all the other stuff that comes with being grown-up.

That's totally okay. I'm not here to make you feel bad or point fingers. My goal is just to nudge you to figure out your special thing and start exploring it, even just a bit. I'm not suggesting you should quit your job or turn your family's life upside down. I'm simply saying it's time to come out of hiding. Begin to gently, consciously connect with your passion, step by step.

Don't worry if you're not quite sure what your thing is yet. That's all part of the journey. That's why it's this big, unspoken dream.

Start now. No more keeping it to yourself. Remember, every great artwork, groundbreaking invention, or life-changing idea started as just a thought that was hard to explain. Think of your unspoken dream as a seed. What grows from it could be something that changes the world – and it will definitely change your life.

## The Importance of Picking Goals You Care About

It is much easier to stay in the trenches when you care about your goal. I mean truly care about them.

If you are struggling to accomplish certain goals, it's important to critically assess why they're on your list. Are these goals genuinely important to you, or are they there because you think they should be? An all-too-common example is setting goals based on societal expectations, like owning a big house or a new car, just to keep up with others. Your goals should be based on what's meaningful to you, not based on external pressures.

We don't set goals just for the sake of it. We set them to grow and to feel better about who we are. Ignoring your past experiences can lead to future disappointments. By understanding and learning from your past, you can set more authentic and personally significant goals.

## How to Achieve Your Goals and Dream

### What to Do

You have set a goal. Say, you want to publish a book. How would you go about doing it?

There is a common trait in people who are achievers: once they identify the obstacles in their path, they take a very specific type of step to start overcoming them – a micro-action. After setting a big goal, they focus on the smallest possible action that nudges them closer to it.

For instance, a friend of mine wanted to publish a book traditionally. The biggest hurdle? She didn't have a publisher. To attract a publisher, you usually need an agent. And to get an agent, you must send what's known as a query letter.

(Notice how we're breaking down a huge challenge into smaller, more manageable steps?)

But the first task was to figure out which agents to contact. Here's what she did: she visited a bookstore, picked up a cookbook, and read the acknowledgments. There, she found the name of an agent the author thanked. That was her micro-action: a simple trip to the bookstore. After noting down one agent's name, the next small step was to look at another cookbook. She continued this process with every cookbook she could, eventually compiling a list of agents.

This story shows the power of micro-actions: starting with something as straightforward as a bookstore visit can set off a chain of steps towards a larger goal.

So, look at your goal. And then. Cut. Cut. Cut. Until you find the doable action. And then you find the next micro-action. And then another one.

## Rather than Resolution, Make a Plan

Creating a plan is more effective than just setting a resolution. Having a goal is a great start, but the real question is how to achieve it.

For instance, if your goal is to earn more money, you need to outline the specific steps to make that happen. How much extra income do you need? If you're employed, could you work overtime or aim for a promotion? Perhaps learning new skills or further education is necessary. Dissecting your goal into smaller, actionable steps makes it more achievable.

A detailed plan increases your chances of success. This idea is supported by research in habit formation. For instance, a study found that people who scheduled their flu shots by noting down the date and time were more likely to get vaccinated than those who just received a reminder.

Additionally, a good plan involves anticipating potential obstacles. People who change successfully often predict where they might face challenges and prepare a strategy to overcome those challenges.

So, sit down, and write down your microactions, your potential obstacles, your options, and your solutions. Be as detailed as possible.

**Reduce Friction**

Goals and dreams are achieved by doing mundane things every single day. The finish line might be fancy. But the work in the gym is very repetitive.

So, how do we stick to our goals?

The main obstacle to achieving your goals is something called friction. To reduce friction, you either remove a hurdle or create a strategy that simplifies a task. Making your goal easier to reach increases your chances of success.

Friction usually appears in three ways: distance, time, and effort. For example, if you live far from your gym or a preferred walking path, chances are you won't go as often. (Research shows that people living over 5 miles from a gym tend to visit only once a month, whereas those within 3.7 miles go about five times a month or more.) Time limitations also hinder new healthy habits. With a packed schedule, finding time for activities like meditation or exercise is tough. Additionally, tasks requiring a lot of effort, such as cooking healthy meals in a chaotic kitchen, are often avoided. If you could create a quick meditation routine of five minutes a day, or you would organize your kitchen, so that you know where everything is, you would reduce friction.

Now, achieving goals, as much as it requires doing certain things, it also involves not doing certain things. For instance, if your goal is increasing muscle muscle, it requires lifting weights, but it also requires not eating certain foods.

If you want to break habits or tendencies, adding friction is the best way. One study demonstrated that making elevator doors close slower by 26 seconds encouraged more people to use the stairs. Similarly, removing vending machines from schools makes it more difficult for students to grab unhealthy snacks or sugary drinks.

So if you want to make a habit, reduce friction i.e. make it easy. If you want to break it, add friction.

## De-Risk Your Goals and Dreams

Deciding to become a professional musician just because your friends love your music might need a second thought.

It's been your lifelong dream to make music your career. Maybe you've saved enough to give it a shot. Your friends and family always rave about your talent. And every day, social media seems to encourage you to follow your passion.

So it feels like the right time to dive in, doesn't it? Maybe invest all your savings into recording an album or setting up a studio.

But pause for a moment. What if your music career doesn't take off?

Perhaps there's a smarter way to pursue this dream. Yes, your inner circle loves your music. That might mean others will too. But that's still a guess.

Why not test it first?

1. Gauge reactions from a broader audience. Play at local venues or open mics where you're not known. Perform your best songs and see how the audience responds. Don't ask directly if you should go pro; just observe their

engagement.

2. Test the market value of your music. Maybe organize a small concert with an entry fee. See how many tickets you sell and watch the audience's reaction. If it's positive, that's a good sign.

3. Start small. Consider releasing your music online or playing at smaller, less expensive venues. If your music resonates, it'll gain traction on platforms like YouTube or Spotify. You don't need a major label deal right away.

Consider growing your dream step by step, driven by real demand, not just your hopes.

Going all-in might look heroic and make a great story, but if it fails, it can be devastating.

There's a safer route: make a hypothesis, test it on a small scale, learn, and iterate. This is how you minimize the risks of a big dream.

## Find Your Whys

Attaching a "why" to every goal can make achieving them much easier and more significant. When your goal is connected to a deeper reason, a few things tend to happen:

1. You'll find yourself more focused on the goal, avoiding distractions or tasks that don't help you reach your desired outcome.

2. It becomes easier to plan, understand, and explain your ideas because you're focused on why you want to achieve something and its potential impact on you.

3. Decisions become more straightforward as your choices are driven by a clear purpose, helping you prioritize effectively.

4. You start to recognize what's truly important in your personal and professional life, leading to greater clarity and meaning.

## Accept Fear

Do you have an ongoing project you only mention to your closest friends and family? The novel that's "almost done," the website you're about to launch, or that email you're about to send your boss to quit your job for freelancing (you're just about to click 'send').

So, what's holding you back?

If you're like me, you work hard, get really close, and then, just as you're about to finish, you hit a snag. And then another.

"What should the logo look like?"

"I can't find a publisher."

"Maybe it needs one more edit."

"Which font is right?"

We pour years into these big dreams. We give our all to reach 85, 90, even 95 percent completion. Then, suddenly, we find ourselves buried in books about font science at the library.

I'm not talking about the hurdles of starting something new. That's a whole other story.

I'm referring to those moments when the finish line is in sight. Here's the thing: it's not about the fonts or the minor details. It's fear.

Fear is the number one thing that stands in the way of our goals and dreams.

The bad news is there is no way around it.

The good news is you can move forward despite it because you see your heroes, those authors, chefs, or entrepreneurs. They feel fear just like you. Some even more than you. Adele, for instance, would throw up backstage from anxiety.

Our own work, when we judge it, never seems finished or good enough. It's not because we're perfectionists. It's because we're afraid. Afraid that no one will like it, afraid it won't succeed, afraid of feeling embarrassed.

What we often do is pick a roadblock and hide behind it. Isn't that interesting? It's like when we were kids, using monsters in our closets as an excuse to hide from our fears.

But let's be clear: being scared isn't the problem. Fear is human, normal, and totally okay. The issue is when our fears stop us from making that big jump from wanting to do something to actually doing it.

Once we realize why we're always stuck at 90 percent, we can start moving towards 100 percent. It's not about a specific roadblock. Now it's about asking, "How do I handle fear?"

That's a far more important question than "What font should I use?" and it's a question that's much more interesting to explore.

**Get an accountability partner**

1. Define "Your Goal." Remember, it's essential that you choose your goal. Ignore the latest trends or pressures from work, friends, or family. It's your decision, based on what you truly want to achieve.

2. Find a trustworthy, close friend and confide Your Goal to them. Make a commitment to accomplish a specific task related to Your Goal within the next week.

3. After the week, meet up with your friend. They should ask if you completed your goal. If you did, celebrate with a high-five. If you didn't, give him $20, $50, or $100.

4. Repeat these steps regularly.

**Cultivate Self Confidence**

Confidence is essential for action. A lack of confidence can stifle efforts before they even begin or disrupt them in progress. For example, if you believe you can get your dream job by applying, you have a better chance of success. But if you don't believe in your ability and therefore don't apply, you'll certainly not achieve this goal. Self-confidence doesn't inherently improve your skills, but it is vital for taking the steps needed to reach your aspirations.

Building self-confidence really comes down to changing how you see yourself. Your self-perception. Here's how you can do that:

### Never be Ashamed About Anything that is Part of Your Life

Being extremely honest with yourself and others is a practical way to build confidence daily. For instance, if you hesitate or feel inclined to hide something when asked about your hobbies or job, that's a sign that you are ashamed. If you have noticed, people who are confident rarely get embarrassed.

This doesn't mean you should share everything with everyone. Discuss specific hobbies with friends who share them and keep work topics for professional settings. The important thing is to not be ashamed of anything that is part of your life. When you stop hiding aspects of yourself, your confidence grows.

## Work Out Regularly

People often start exercising for physical benefits, but it's also a great way to boost self-confidence. Regular exercise has been shown to improve mood and aid mental health. Maintaining a workout routine is a personal victory, and seeing consistent commitment through can make you feel more confident.

And, let's be honest, when you look better you feel more confident.

## Embrace Discomfort

Actively stepping out of your comfort zone is uncomfortable by nature, but it's essential for developing confidence. Confidence stems from being comfortable in situations that would typically be challenging. By gradually expanding your comfort zone, you'll find yourself becoming more adaptable in various scenarios.

This might involve significant changes like a new job or confronting difficult issues, or it could be smaller steps like engaging in new social interactions if you're introverted, or experimenting with different foods. The objective is to consistently push your boundaries.

## Loving the Process

Finding joy in the journey towards your goal is vital for keeping up your motivation. People often go through stages: the tough grind of work, then worry about failing, and finally enjoyment. However, it's key to find joy in the work itself, not just wait for the end. Think about how you feel when you imagine pursuing your goal. If you feel stressed, it might not be the right goal or the right time. But if you feel interested and open, that's a great sign.

The journey won't always feel great, so recognizing and celebrating small wins along the way is important. These little successes keep you going. Remember, it's often easier to handle small steps than big leaps. Keeping yourself motivated through self-recognition really helps.

When you do achieve your goal, you might find that the process was the real reward. Every day of effort and progress is what leads to success. The goal is like a victory lap for all your hard work.

## Have a Growth Mindset

A growth mindset is like looking at life as an endless classroom, where every challenge is a new lesson and every failure a chance to learn. It's believing that with effort and persistence, you can get better at anything, whether it's a skill, a subject, or a hobby.

Imagine a kid learning to ride a bike. At first, they fall a lot, and it's frustrating. With a fixed mindset, they might think, "I'm just not good at this," and give up. But with a growth mindset, they'd think, "I'm not good at this yet, but I can learn." So, they keep trying, learning from each fall, until one day, they're riding without even thinking about it.

It's like this in all areas of life. Take a musician learning a new piece. It's tough, and there are parts they can't play yet. In a growth mindset, instead of saying, "I can't do this," they think, "I can't do this yet." They practice those hard parts, slowly at first, then faster, until they can play the whole piece.

This mindset isn't just about saying you can improve; it's about really believing it and acting on it. It means when you get a bad grade or a project at work doesn't go well, instead of feeling defeated, you think about what went wrong and how you can do better next time. You ask for feedback, you try different strategies, and you don't give up.

People with a growth mindset don't see effort as a bad thing. They don't think needing to work hard at something means they're not smart or talented. Instead, they see effort as the way to get smarter and more talented. They're not afraid of challenges or mistakes; they welcome them as chances to grow.

So, a growth mindset is about more than just trying hard. It's about loving learning, being resilient in the face of setbacks, and understanding that the journey to getting better at anything is often slow and full of ups and downs. It's about seeing potential and possibility in yourself, no matter where you're starting from.

## Have Self Compassion

Take a blank sheet of paper and draw a line down the middle. First, think about the last time you saw someone else fail. It might be hard to remember. Once you do, write down a few words on the left side of the paper about how their failure made you think of them.

Next, think about your own last failure. This memory might come more quickly. On the right side, write a few words describing how that failure made you feel about yourself.

Now, compare both sides. Often, two things happen:

1. Remembering someone else's failure might be difficult, but recalling your own could bring a flood of memories.
2. On the left side, you might have words like 'compassion,' 'courage,' and 'bravery' for the other person. On the right, words like 'shame' and 'stupidity' for yourself.

It's interesting, isn't it? We often admire others for their attempts, even if they fail, but harshly criticize ourselves for the same. We also tend to quickly forgive and forget others' mistakes while clinging to our own for much longer.

Self-compassion should be a big part of the diet of a goal-seeker, lest you turn into a goal-avoider.

Before We Get Started...

Remember, mindfulness journaling is a personal practice, and these questions are meant to guide and inspire you. Feel free to adapt and modify them to suit your needs and preferences. Explore, reflect, and embrace the opportunity to deepen your self-awareness and cultivate a sense of inner peace.

Date ___ / ___ / ___: S   M   T   W   Th   F   S

**I feel:**
(please circle)

because _____   because _____   because _____   because _____   because _____
_____   _____   _____   _____   _____

## Today I Am Grateful For

1. _____
2. _____
3. _____

What could help transform today into a remarkable day?

## Reflective Writing

What are your biggest goals and dreams?

_____

_____

_____

_____

_____

_____

_____

_____

# What is the first step you should take in setting a personal goal?

a) Identify your strengths and weaknesses
b) Write down your goal in detail
c) Share your goal with a friend or family member
d) Ensure the goal is realistic and achievable

All Are Correct - Choose The Response You Feel Is Most Important To Remember

Date ___ / ___ / ___ : S   M   T   W   Th   F   S

I feel:
(please circle)

because _____    because _____    because _____    because _____    because _____

## Today I Am Grateful For

1. _____
2. _____
3. _____

What could help transform today into a remarkable day?

## Reflective Writing

What have you done to move closer to achieving them?

_____

_____

_____

_____

_____

_____

_____

# What is the best way to stay motivated towards achieving your goals?

a) Reward yourself for every small accomplishment
b) Keep your goals to yourself
c) Focus on the end result, not the process
d) Set a strict timeline for achieving your goals

All Are Correct - Choose The Response You Feel Is Most Important To Remember

Date ___ / ___ / ___ : S M T W Th F S

**I feel:**
(please circle)

because    because    because    because    because

_____ _____ _____ _____ _____

_____ _____ _____ _____ _____

## Today I Am Grateful For

1. _____
2. _____
3. _____

What could help transform today into a remarkable day?

_____

## Reflective Writing

What do you think is holding you back from
achieving them?

_____

_____

_____

_____

_____

_____

_____

# What is the benefit of setting specific and measurable goals?

a) It makes it easier to track progress
b) It allows for flexibility in changing goals
c) It ensures your goals are achievable
d) It eliminates the need for a timeline

All Are Correct - Choose The Response You Feel Is Most Important To Remember

Date ___ / ___ / ___ : S   M   T   W   Th   F   S

I feel:
(please circle)

because   because   because   because   because
_____   _____   _____   _____   _____
_____   _____   _____   _____   _____

## Today I Am Grateful For

1. _____
2. _____
3. _____

What could help transform today into a remarkable day?

## Reflective Writing

How do you stay motivated when it comes to your goals and dreams?

_____

_____

_____

_____

_____

_____

# What is a common reason for not achieving personal goals?

a) Lack of motivation
b) Too many distractions
c) Unrealistic expectations
d) Lack of support from others

All Are Correct - Choose The Response You Feel Is Most Important
To Remember

Date ___ / ___ / ___ : S   M   T   W   Th   F   S

**I feel:**
(please circle)

because _____   because _____   because _____   because _____   because _____

## Today I Am Grateful For

1. _____
2. _____
3. _____

What could help transform today into a remarkable day?

## Reflective Writing

What are your short-term, mid-term, and long-term goals?

_____

_____

_____

_____

_____

_____

_____

# How can you overcome obstacles when working towards your goals?

a) Give up and set new goals

b) Tackle one obstacle at a time

c) Ignore the obstacles and continue anyway

d) Ask for help from family or friends

All Are Correct - Choose The Response You Feel Is Most Important To Remember

Date ___ / ___ / ___ : S  M  T  W  Th  F  S

I feel:
(please circle)

because _____ _____
because _____ _____
because _____ _____
because _____ _____
because _____ _____

## Today I Am Grateful For

1. _____
2. _____
3. _____

What could help transform today into a remarkable day?

## Reflective Writing

What steps do you need to take to make your
goals and dreams a reality?

_____

_____

_____

_____

_____

_____

_____

## What is the difference between a short-term goal and a long-term goal?

a) Timeframe and level of priority

b) Difficulty and cost

c) Importance and value

d) Type of motivation needed

All Are Correct - Choose The Response You Feel Is Most Important To Remember

Date ___ / ___ / ___ : **S M T W Th F S**

**I feel:**
(please circle)

because _____ because _____ because _____ because _____ because _____
_____ _____ _____ _____ _____

## Today I Am Grateful For

1. _____
2. _____
3. _____

What could help transform today into a remarkable day?

## Reflective Writing

What resources do you need to achieve your goals and dreams?

_____

_____

_____

_____

_____

_____

# Which of the following can help in setting and achieving realistic goals?

a) Seeking guidance from a mentor or coach
b) Setting goals that require minimal effort
c) Setting goals based on what others are doing
d) Setting goals that are easy to achieve

All Are Correct - Choose The Response You Feel Is Most Important To Remember

Date ___ / ___ / ___ : S  M  T  W  Th  F  S

I feel:
(please circle)

because   because   because   because   because

_____  _____  _____  _____  _____

_____  _____  _____  _____  _____

## Today I Am Grateful For

1. _____
2. _____
3. _____

What could help transform today into a remarkable day?

## Reflective Writing

What are the biggest obstacles in the way of achieving your goals and dreams?

_____

_____

_____

_____

_____

_____

_____

# What is a good way to stay accountable for your goals?

a) Keeping your goals a secret
b) Keeping a journal of your progress
c) Focusing on other people's accomplishments
d) Setting unrealistic expectations

All Are Correct - Choose The Response You Feel Is Most Important To Remember

Date \_\_ / \_\_ / \_\_ : S   M   T   W   Th   F   S

I feel:
(please circle)

because   because   because   because   because

_____   _____   _____   _____   _____

_____   _____   _____   _____   _____

## Today I Am Grateful For

1. _____
2. _____
3. _____

What could help transform today into a remarkable day?

## Reflective Writing

What have you learned about yourself by exploring your personal goals and dreams?

_____

_____

_____

_____

_____

_____

# How can visualization help in achieving your goals?

a) It allows you to escape from reality
b) It helps you to set unattainable goals
c) It makes you forget about your goals
d) It keeps you focused and motivated

All Are Correct - Choose The Response You Feel Is Most Important To Remember

45

Date ___ / ___ / ___ : S M T W Th F S

I feel: (please circle)

because _____ because _____ because _____ because _____ because _____

_____ _____ _____ _____ _____

## Today I Am Grateful For

1. _____
2. _____
3. _____

What could help transform today into a remarkable day?

## Reflective Writing

What advice would you give to someone who is trying to achieve their goals and dreams?

_____

_____

_____

_____

_____

_____

_____

**What is the importance of creating a plan for achieving your goals?**

a) It ensures that you only take small steps towards your goal
b) It allows you to easily change your goals
c) It provides a roadmap to success
d) It limits your ability to be creative

All Are Correct - Choose The Response You Feel Is Most Important To Remember

Date ___ / ___ / ___ :  S   M   T   W   Th   F   S

I feel:
(please circle)

because    because    because    because    because
_____    _____    _____    _____    _____
_____    _____    _____    _____    _____

## Today I Am Grateful For

1. _____
2. _____
3. _____

What could help transform today into a remarkable day?

### Reflective Writing

How does your current lifestyle support or hinder your journey towards achieving your goals and dreams?

_____

_____

_____

_____

_____

_____

_____

# What is the best way to handle setbacks when working towards your goals?

a) Give up on the goal entirely
b) Adjust the goal and make it easier
c) Take some time to reflect and reevaluate
d) Ignore the setback and continue as planned

All Are Correct - Choose The Response You Feel Is Most Important To Remember

Date ___ / ___ / ___ : S  M  T  W  Th  F  S

I feel:
(please circle)

because _____ because _____ because _____ because _____ because _____

## Today I Am Grateful For

1. _____
2. _____
3. _____

What could help transform today into a remarkable day?

## Reflective Writing

How do your values and beliefs help you to stay on track with achieving your goals and dreams?

_____

_____

_____

_____

_____

_____

_____

_____

# How can gratitude help in achieving your goals?

a) It makes you more complacent with your current situation
b) It allows you to appreciate the journey towards your goal
c) It distracts you from your goals
d) It makes you lose focus on what you want to achieve

All Are Correct - Choose The Response You Feel Is Most Important To Remember

I feel:
(please circle)

because    because    because    because    because

_____  _____  _____  _____  _____

_____  _____  _____  _____  _____

## Today I Am Grateful For

1. _____
2. _____
3. _____

What could help transform today into a remarkable day?

## Reflective Writing
What strategies do you use to stay focused on
your goals and dreams?

_____

_____

_____

_____

_____

_____

_____

# What is an example of a realistic personal goal?

a) Becoming a millionaire overnight
b) Running a marathon without any training
c) Losing 50 pounds in a week
d) Starting a daily exercise routine

All Are Correct - Choose The Response You Feel Is Most Important To Remember

Date ___ / ___ / ___ : S  M  T  W  Th  F  S

# I feel:
(please circle)

because  because  because  because  because
_____  _____  _____  _____  _____
_____  _____  _____  _____  _____

## Today I Am Grateful For

1. _____
2. _____
3. _____

What could help transform today into a remarkable day?

## Reflective Writing

How do you measure success when it comes to achieving your goals and dreams?

_____

_____

_____

_____

_____

_____

_____

# Why is it important to set goals in different areas of your life?

a) To have a well-rounded life
b) To have more things to focus on
c) To feel overwhelmed and challenged
d) To impress others with your accomplishments

All Are Correct - Choose The Response You Feel Is Most Important To Remember

Date ___ / ___ / ___ : S  M  T  W  Th  F  S

I feel:
(please circle)

because _____ _____

because _____ _____

because _____ _____

because _____ _____

because _____ _____

## Today I Am Grateful For

1. _____
2. _____
3. _____

What could help transform today into a remarkable day?

## Reflective Writing

How can you use the support of others to help you reach your goals and dreams?

_____

_____

_____

_____

_____

_____

_____

# How can writing down your goals help in achieving them?

a) It makes the goals more official
b) It allows you to keep track of your progress
c) It shows others how determined you are
d) It doesn't have any impact on the achievement of the goal

All Are Correct - Choose The Response You Feel Is Most Important To Remember

As we reach the final pages of this journey through "Positive Mindset," I want to extend my heartfelt thanks to you. Your commitment to exploring positivity and its transformative power is not only commendable but a testament to your desire for personal growth and a richer, more fulfilling life experience.

Remember, the journey towards a positive mindset is ongoing and ever-evolving. Each day presents new opportunities to apply these principles, to learn, and to grow. I encourage you to revisit these pages whenever you need a reminder of your incredible potential to foster positivity and resilience in the face of life's challenges.

As we part ways, I leave you with a quote that has been a guiding star in my journey: "The greatest discovery of any generation is that a human can alter his life by altering his attitude."

– William James.

Thank you for allowing me to be a part of your journey. May your path be filled with light, hope, and endless possibilities. Farewell, and may you carry the spirit of positivity with you, today and always.

With gratitude and best wishes,

Sensei Paul David

# Reflective Writing

_____

_____

_____

_____

_____

_____

_____

_____

_____

_____

_____

_____

_____

_____

_____

_____

_____

_____

_____

_____

_____

_____

# The End

As you close the pages of this mindfulness journal, remember that each word you've written is a step on your journey towards self-awareness and inner peace. Embrace the moments of clarity, the revelations, and even the uncertainties you've encountered along the way. Let this journal be a testament to your growth and a reminder that every day offers a new opportunity to be present, to observe, and to appreciate the simple wonders of life. Carry these lessons forward, and may your path be filled with mindful moments and serene reflections. Until we meet again in these pages, be gentle with yourself and stay anchored in the now.

Mindfulness isn't difficult, we just need to remember to do it.

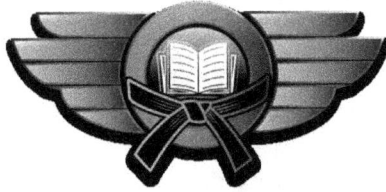

# Thank You!

If you found this book helpful, I would be grateful if you would **post an honest review on Amazon** so this book can reach other supportive readers like you!

All you need to do is digitally flip to the back and leave your review. Or visit amazon.com/author/senseipauldavid click the correct book cover and click on the blue link next to the yellow stars that say, "customer reviews."

## *As always...*
## *It's a great day to be alive!*

# Get/Share Your FREE SSD Mental Health Chronicles at
## www.senseiselfdevelopment.care

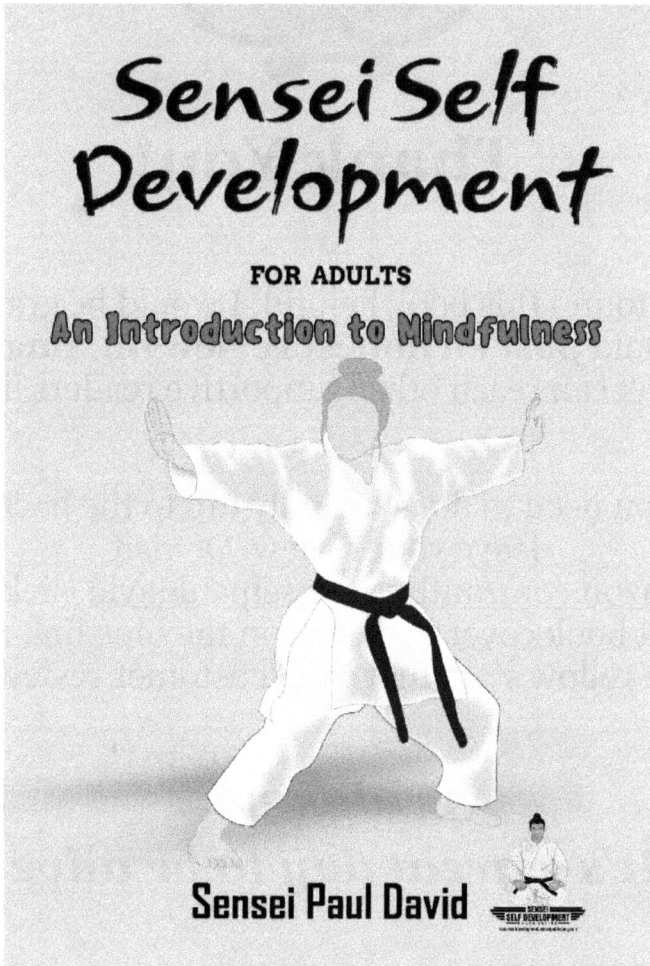

# Sensei Self Development

**FOR ADULTS**

## An Introduction to Mindfulness

## Sensei Paul David

# Check Out The SSD Chronicles
## Series CLICK HERE

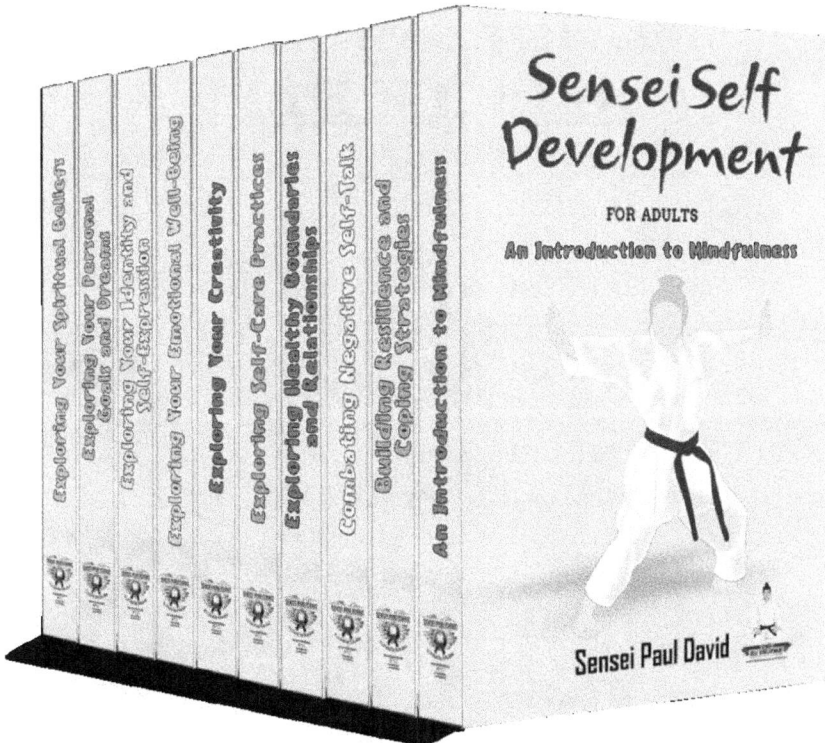

# Get/Share Your FREE All-Ages Mental Health eBook Now at

www.senseiselfdevelopment.com

## Or CLICK HERE

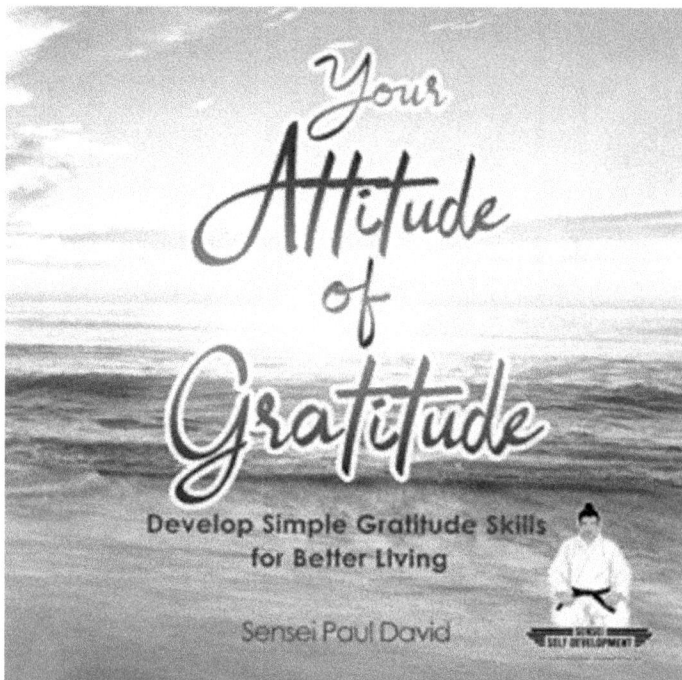

senseiselfdevelopment.com

# Click Another Book In The SSD BOOK SERIES:

senseipublishing.com/SSD_SERIES

## CLICK HERE

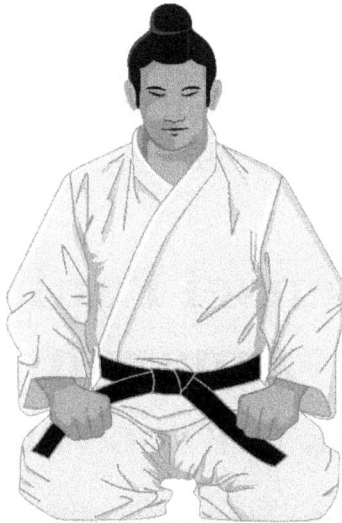

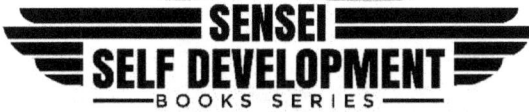

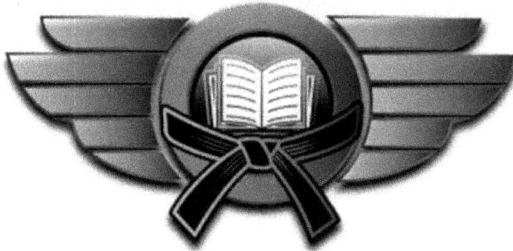

# Join Our Publishing Journey!

If you would like to receive FREE BOOKS, please visit **www.senseipublishing.com**.  Join our newsletter by entering your email address in the pop-up box

# Follow Sensei Paul David on Amazon

## CLICK THE LOGO BELOW

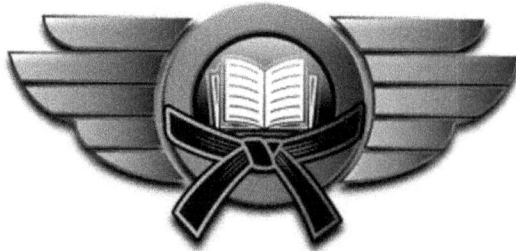

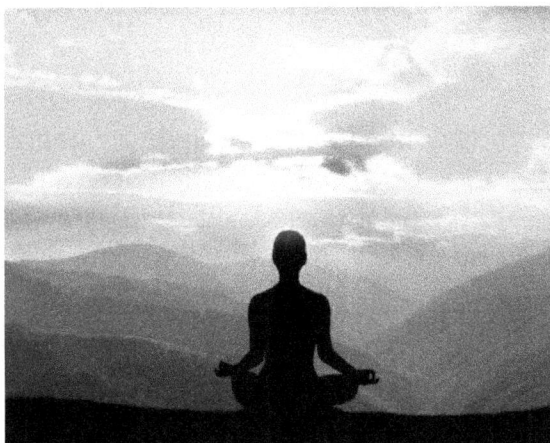

**FREE BONUS!!!**
**Experience Over 25 FREE Engaging Guided Meditations!**

Prized Skills & Practices for Adults & Kids. Help Restore Deep-Sleep, Lower Stress, Improve Posture, Navigate Uncertainty & More.

Download the Free Insight Timer App and click the link below:
**http://insig.ht/sensei_paul**

# About Sensei Publishing

Sensei Publishing commits itself to helping people of all ages transform into better versions of themselves by providing high-quality and research-based self-development books with an emphasis on mental health and guided meditations. Sensei Publishing offers well-written e-books, audiobooks, paperbacks and online courses that simplify complicated but practical topics in line with its mission to inspire people towards positive transformation.

It's a great day to be alive!

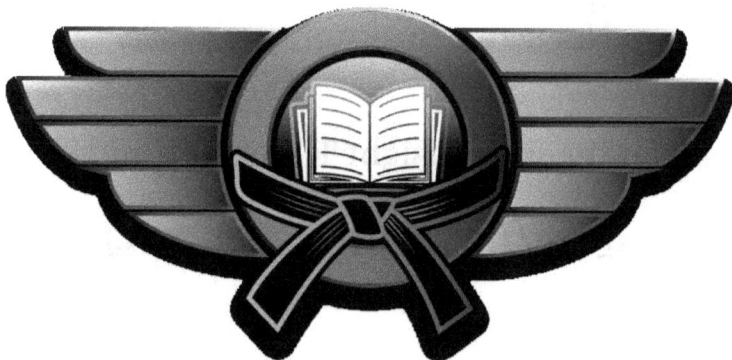

# About the Author

I create simple & transformative eBooks & Guided Meditations for Adults & Children proven to help navigate uncertainty, solve niche problems & bring families closer together.

I'm a former finance project manager, private pilot, jiu-jitsu instructor, musician & former University of Toronto Fitness Trainer.  I prefer a science-based approach to focus on these & other areas in my life to stay humble & hungry to evolve. I hope you enjoy my work and I'd love to hear your feedback.

- It's a great day to be alive!

Sensei Paul David

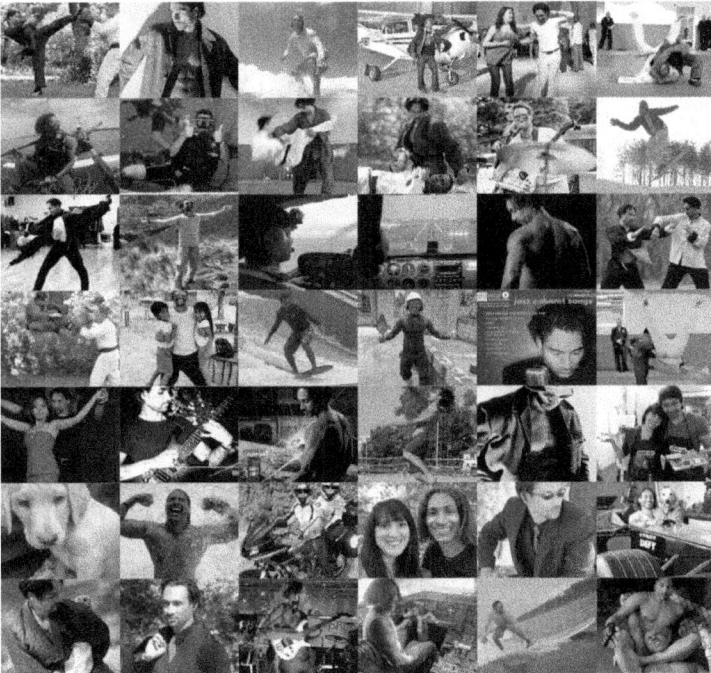

Scan & Follow/Like/Subscribe: Facebook, Instagram,
YouTube: @senseipublishing

Scan using your phone/iPad camera for Social Media
Visit us at www.senseipublishing.com and sign up for our
newsletter to learn more about our exciting books and to
experience our FREE Guided Meditations for Kids & Adults.